BEYOND SHAMPOO

A Guide to Healthy Hair Growth and Maintenance

By Kira Rodriguez

Copyright © 2023

DISCLAIMER

The information contained in this hair care book is intended for educational purposes only. The reader should be aware that individual results may vary, and the information in this book is not a substitute for professional medical advice, diagnosis, or treatment. The information in this book is based on the author's personal experiences, research, and knowledge, and it is not intended to diagnose, treat, cure, or prevent any disease.

TABLE OF CONTENTS

CHAPTER 1

INTRODUCTION

The key to maintaining healthy hair is an essential goal for many people, regardless of their hair type, length, or texture. In order to achieve this goal, there are several things you can do to take care of your hair. For example, it's important to avoid excessive heat, chemicals, and styling tools that can weaken your hair and make it more prone to damage. Instead, focus on using natural and nourishing hair care products, such as shampoo and conditioner that's suited to your hair type.

The process of hair growth starts with small pockets in the skin known as follicles, which contain blood vessels and nourishing proteins that our body uses to grow our hair. As more cells are generated, hair starts to grow in length and pushes through the skin. Hair is made up of a hard protein called keratin, which makes it look like dead matter on the surface, and the further it grows away from the scalp, the drier it can become.

Genetics play a major role in determining how quickly hair grows, but there are other factors that can impact hair growth as well. For example, a diet that's rich in protein and nutrients can help to promote healthy hair growth.

Hormones, such as those associated with pregnancy or menopause, can also impact hair growth. To keep your hair healthy and strong, it's important to take a proactive approach to hair care. This means using the right products for your hair type, and avoiding excessive manipulation and styling that can cause damage to your hair. Protecting your hair from weather elements, such as the sun's UV rays and harsh winds during the winter months, is also important in preventing damage and promoting healthy hair.

In summary, taking care of your hair is essential for healthy growth and appearance, regardless of your hair type.

Understanding the process of hair growth, factors that impact growth, and taking steps to protect your hair can help you achieve and maintain healthy, strong, and beautiful hair.

CHAPTER 2

KNOW YOUR HAIR

Hair Density

The average human scalp contains approximately 100,000 hair follicles, although this number can vary based on several factors such as age, gender, and ethnicity. Hair density can also vary, and is typically classified as thick, medium, or thin. Thick hair density is characterized by closely packed hair that makes it difficult to see the scalp. Medium hair density means that hair is less closely packed, allowing some scalp to be visible. Finally, thin hair density refers to hair that is widely spaced apart, which can make the scalp more visible and give the impression of thinner hair.

Hair Texture

Hair texture is determined by the diameter of each individual hair strand, and it can be classified into three main categories: fine, medium, and coarse.

Fine hair has a smaller diameter than medium or coarse hair. It is very easy to process and style, but it can also be prone to damage from chemical treatments like coloring, perming, and relaxing due to its delicate nature. Fine hair can also lack volume and body, and may require special products and styling techniques to add texture and fullness.

Medium hair has a diameter that falls between fine and coarse hair. It is the most common hair type, and is generally considered to be the most versatile. Medium hair can be styled in a variety of ways and can handle a range of different hair products, from lightweight mousses to heavy gels. It may require some extra care and conditioning to keep it healthy and manageable, but overall it is a fairly low-maintenance hair type.

Coarse hair has a larger diameter than fine or medium hair. It tends to be more resistant to chemical treatments like coloring and perming because it has more substance and texture. However, coarse hair can be more difficult to style and may require extra moisture and conditioning to keep it looking healthy and shiny. Coarse hair also tends to be more prone to frizz and may require specialized hair products and styling techniques to keep it under control.

Hair Porosity

Porosity refers to the hair's ability to absorb and retain moisture, and can be categorized into three main categories:

Low porosity hair has a tightly closed cuticle layer, which makes it difficult for moisture to penetrate the hair shaft.

As a result, low porosity hair can be resistant to chemical treatments and may require special techniques to fully saturate it with water and products.

Average porosity hair has a slightly raised cuticle layer, which allows moisture and product to enter the hair shaft easily, while still maintaining good moisture retention. This is the most common type of hair porosity.

High porosity hair has a damaged or porous cuticle layer, which causes the hair to absorb moisture quickly but also release it quickly. This type of hair is often dry, brittle, and prone to breakage. High porosity hair can benefit from regular deep conditioning and protein treatments to help strengthen the hair shaft and reduce breakage. Understanding the porosity of your hair can be helpful when choosing hair products and determining the best hair care routine for your hair type.

Hair Elasticity

Hair elasticity is the ability of hair to stretch and contract without breaking, and it can be likened to the elasticity of a rubber band.

To test hair elasticity, stylists can pull a wet strand of hair and see if it stretches and returns to its original form without breaking.

Hair with normal elasticity can stretch up to 20% of its natural length when dry and up to 50% when wet without breaking. Good elasticity is a sign of healthy hair that can handle styling without damage.

Low hair elasticity, on the other hand, is marked by breakage, difficulty in holding curls, and a lack of stretch. Factors such as excessive heat styling, over-processing with chemicals, and inadequate moisture can contribute to low hair elasticity. Hair with low elasticity requires extra care and attention to enhance its strength and flexibility.

In summary, hair elasticity is important for healthy hair and allows for styling without causing damage. Testing hair elasticity is easy for stylists, and low elasticity can be addressed with appropriate hair care practices.

Hair subcategory

There are various ways to categorize hair types, such as curl pattern and texture. Here are some common types and their characteristics:

Type 1:

1A: Hair is soft and lacks curl, making it difficult to hold a curl. It tends to have more volume instead.

1B: Hair is straight and lacks curl, but has more body and volume.

1C: Hair is straight and coarse, and does not hold a curl well.

Type 2:

2A: Hair has a slight wave that resembles the letter "S". It is coarse in texture.

2B: Hair has a definite wave and tends to be frizzy.

2C: Hair is very frizzy and has thick waves. It is the coarsest of the Type 2 category.

Type 3:

3A: Hair has loose curls that are about the same diameter as sidewalk chalk.

3B: Hair has medium-sized curls that are about the same diameter as a Sharpie marker.

3C: Hair has tight corkscrew curls that are about the same diameter as a pencil.

Type 4:

4A: Hair has tight, defined curls that resemble the letter "S". It is prone to dryness, frizz, and can appear slightly dull without product.

4B: Hair has a zigzag pattern that looks like the letter "Z". It has a fluffier texture than Type 4A and is susceptible to dryness and breakage.

4C: Hair has a tightly coiled, zigzag pattern that can appear uneven and does not have a clear curl pattern. It is the most fragile of the Type 4 category.

CHAPTER 3

WASH DAY GUIDE

A wash day guide may include the following steps:

1.Pre-poo:

- ☐ Divide hair into 4 sections

- ☐ Apply an oil such as coconut or olive oil to each section

- ☐ Cover hair with a plastic cap and leave it for at least 30 minutes

- ☐ Rinse out the oil

2.Shampoo (or co-wash):

- ☐ Use a sulfate-free shampoo and wash hair in sections

- ☐ Avoid being too rough when washing

- ☐ Concentrate on your roots, where there may be product buildup

☐ Rinse hair thoroughly

3. Conditioner:

☐ Apply a sulfate-free conditioner to each section

☐ Focus on your ends

☐ Detangle hair using a wide-tooth comb

☐ Rinse out the conditioner

4. Deep Conditioner:

☐ Apply a deep conditioner to each section and cover hair for at least 30 minutes

☐ Rinse out the conditioner with normal water

5. Moisturize:

☐ Moisturize hair when it's damp

☐ Apply a leave-in conditioner and concentrate on your ends

- [] Use oil to seal in the moisture

- [] Avoid piling too many products on your hair

6. Style:

- [] Opt for a protective style

- [] Avoid styles that pull too much on your edges, as excessive tension can cause breakage.

CHAPTER 4

SOME DIY HAIR MASKS

Using natural ingredients that are commonly found at home, DIY hair masks are a convenient way to nourish and strengthen your hair. Here are some popular DIY hair masks:

Repairing: Mix one tablespoon of coconut oil with one tablespoon of honey, heat it up a little, apply it to the hair, leave it on for 30 minutes, then shampoo and condition the hair.

Hair growth: Mix one tablespoon of coconut oil with one teaspoon of cinnamon, apply it to the scalp, massage it in, leave it on for 30 minutes, then shampoo and condition the hair.

Dry hair: Mix two tablespoons of brown sugar with one tablespoon of olive oil, apply it to the hair, leave it on for 15-20 minutes, then shampoo and condition the hair.

Frizzy hair: Mix banana, yogurt, and honey, apply it to the hair, leave it on for 30-45 minutes, then shampoo and condition the hair.

Damaged hair: Mash one avocado in a bowl, add two eggs, one tablespoon of honey, and one tablespoon of coconut oil, mix well, apply it to the hair, leave it on for 30 minutes, then shampoo and condition the hair.

Guava leaves: Boil fresh guava leaves in water, let it cool, strain the leaves, apply it to the hair and scalp, leave it on for 30 minutes, then rinse and proceed with your routine.

Dandruff: Mix warm coconut oil and lemon juice, apply it to the scalp and hair, leave it on for 30 minutes, then shampoo and condition the hair. Repeat consistently until dandruff is gone.

__Hair growth__: Mix a few drops of rosemary oil with coconut oil, and use it for a scalp massage.

__Thinning hair or hair loss on edges:__ Combine castor oil with a few drops of tea tree oil and/or peppermint oil, and apply it twice daily for results.

__Banana and Honey Mask:__ Combine one mashed ripe banana with two tablespoons of honey. Apply the mixture to your hair, leave it on for 30 minutes, and then rinse it out with shampoo and conditioner.

__Egg and Olive Oil Mask:__ Beat one egg with two tablespoons of olive oil and apply it to your hair. Leave it on for 20-30 minutes, and then rinse it out with shampoo and conditioner.

__Avocado and Coconut Oil Mask:__ Mash one ripe avocado and mix it with two tablespoons of coconut oil. Apply it to your hair, leave it on for 30 minutes, and then rinse it out with shampoo and conditioner.

Yogurt and Lemon Juice Mask: Mix half a cup of plain yogurt with two tablespoons of lemon juice. Apply the mixture to your hair, leave it on for 30 minutes, and then rinse it out with shampoo and conditioner.

Apple Cider Vinegar and Honey Mask: Mix two tablespoons of apple cider vinegar with one tablespoon of honey. Apply the mixture to your hair, leave it on for 20-30 minutes, and then rinse it out with shampoo and conditioner.

While these DIY hair masks can help improve the condition of your hair, it's important to remember that everyone's hair is different. If you have any concerns or allergies, it's best to consult with a healthcare professional before trying any new hair masks.

CHAPTER 5

HANDLING NATURAL HAIR

Maintaining natural hair can require specific techniques and products to keep it healthy and looking its best. Below are some tips for handling natural hair:

- Keep your hair moisturized: Natural hair often lacks moisture, so it's crucial to keep it hydrated. You can use a leave-in conditioner or oil to help lock in moisture.

- Detangle gently: To avoid hair breakage, detangle your hair gently with your fingers or a wide-tooth comb. Start from the ends and work your way up to the roots.

- Protect your hair while sleeping: When you sleep, use a silk or satin headscarf or pillowcase to prevent breakage and retain moisture in your hair.

- [] Use suitable hair products: Look for hair products that are formulated specifically for natural hair. Avoid using products containing alcohol or sulfates, which can dry out your hair.

- [] Minimize heat styling: Applying heat to your hair frequently can damage it. If you must heat-style, use a heat protectant spray and set the heat to low.

- [] Trim your hair regularly: To keep your hair looking healthy, trim it regularly to prevent split ends and breakage.

- [] Experiment with different styles: Natural hair is versatile, so you can try various styles such as braids, twists, buns, or updo.

- [] Understand what your hair needs to thrive; proper nutrition, adequate moisture, proper handling.

- Hair care routine: Create a simple hair care routine that is within budget and fits well with lifestyle. Test out the hair care routine and if need be, make adjustments. It only gets better with time and patience. And be consistent with your hair care routine.

- Hair Combing: Don't comb dry hair because it will increase the rate of breakage, comb on moist hair. Use a wide tooth comb and always keep them clean. Comb hair in sections starting from the tips of hair to the roots (scalp).

- Detangle hair completely before going to a salon.

- Hair style: Go for protective hairstyles (low manipulation styles) Avoid styles that pull too much on your hair strands.

☐ Protect hair during sleep: Use satin bonnet to bed or satin pillowcase.

☐ Scalp massage: Scalp massage can increase blood circulation to the hair follicles, which can help promote hair growth.

☐ Incorporate one new product at a time to determine its effectiveness.

☐ Journaling can help you keep track of your hair goals and progress.

☐ Love your hair for everything and everything it is not.

☐ Undo tight ponytails or other restrictive banding to prevent stress on the hairline.

It's important to note that every individual's hair is different, and what works for one person may not work for another. Be patient, try different techniques, and find what works best for your natural hair.

CHAPTER 6

SAMPLE OF HAIR REGIMEN

A hair regimen is essentially a set of practices and routines that you establish to take care of your hair. By following a proper hair regimen, you can help maintain healthy hair, encourage growth, and prevent damage.

This can involve using appropriate products for your hair type, creating a consistent washing and conditioning routine, taking steps to protect your hair from heat and environmental damage, and practicing other healthy hair habits like regular trims and avoiding hairstyles that can cause breakage. By making a habit of following a hair regimen, you can help keep your hair looking and feeling its best.

Establishing an effective and consistent hair care routine:

Daily hair care routine

A daily hair care routine typically consists of a set of habits and practices that help to keep your hair healthy and looking its best. One important aspect of this routine is to maintain proper moisture levels in the hair by using products like leave-in conditioners, oils, and serums. Additionally, it's crucial to protect your hair from damage and breakage while sleeping, which can be achieved by wearing a satin bonnet or scarf.

It's important to choose products that are appropriate for your hair type and establish a consistent routine that works well with your schedule. While it may not always be possible to moisturize your hair every day, it's recommended to do so every 2-3 days to help maintain healthy hair.

Other essential aspects of a daily hair care routine may include washing and conditioning your hair regularly, using appropriate styling products and tools, and protecting your hair from environmental factors like heat and the sun. By establishing a daily hair care routine, you can help keep your hair strong, healthy, and looking great.

Weekly hair care routine

Maintaining a weekly hair care routine is essential for promoting healthy hair. Washing your hair daily with shampoo can cause dryness and damage, so it is recommended to limit shampooing to once a week or twice a month. Alternatively, you can use cowashing, which involves washing your hair with conditioner only, in between shampoos.

Along with washing your hair, a weekly hair care routine should also include conditioning and deep conditioning treatments to provide your hair with the nourishment it needs.

Using leave-in conditioners or hair masks can help to hydrate and moisturize your hair, which can prevent dryness and damage. It's also important to take steps to protect your hair from heat and environmental factors, such as using a heat protectant spray or wearing a hat. Regular trimming to get rid of split ends can also help keep your hair healthy and prevent further damage. By establishing a consistent weekly hair care routine, you can help keep your hair healthy, strong, and looking its best.

Monthly hair care routine

A monthly hair care routine typically involves special treatments that can provide intensive nourishment and hydration to your hair. These treatments are designed to promote healthy hair growth and include options like rice water treatments, the inversion method, and herbal treatments. One of the most popular treatments is the rice water treatment, which involves soaking rice in water and using the resulting liquid to rinse your hair.

This treatment is believed to strengthen the hair, improve its elasticity, and promote growth. Another option is the inversion method, which involves hanging your head upside down for a period of time each day to increase blood flow to the scalp and promote hair growth. Herbal treatments, such as henna, can also be beneficial for your hair as they can help to strengthen and condition it, as well as promote growth.

Incorporating these special treatments into a monthly hair care routine can help give your hair the extra care it needs to stay healthy and looking its best. To achieve the best results, it's important to choose treatments that are appropriate for your hair type and needs, and to be consistent with your routine.

CONSIDER THE FOLLOWING WHEN CREATING A REGIMEN

Proper diet and nutrition

This is very important to hair growth. The body needs to be healthy in order to grow healthy hair, therefore, ensure the proper intake of the right vitamins, nutrients, minerals, and other supplements.

Pre-poo natural hair before shampooing

This is a hair treatment done in preparing the hair before shampooing. The main purpose of pre-poo is to ensure the hair is well prepared for the shampooing process. As it protects hair from the harsh and stripping nature of shampoo. And it helps make detangling easier, add moisture, and also improves manageability.

Condition hair after shampooing

Hair conditioning should be done every time one shampoos the hair. It works on the outside by softening the hair and minimizing static. As it improves the manageability by reducing friction between the hair strands making the hair smooth and strong.

Moisturize and seal moisture using LOC/LCO method

This is to prevent hair from losing the moisture that one have worked so hard for, so one will need to seal in the moisture properly. Hair moisturizing can simply be done by applying hair with water, or a leave-in conditioner then adding an oil and following with a cream, this is called the LOC method. While the LCO method, liquid before cream, then oil.

The liquid is the moisture, talking or moisture, water is moisture. And to retain that, that is where oil and cream come in. Oil helps the hair hold on to water molecules, like coconut oil, avocado oil, olive oil, etc.

They increase the hair's capability to hold on to water molecules. Cream locks in moisture. Shea butter or mango butter can be used as cream in cases of extremely dry hair. The best sealant includes castor oil, grape seed oil and jojoba oil.

Wear hair in protective styles

Select a hairstyle that will not only look good, but is also protective such as braids, twists, weaved hairstyles etc. If you leave a protective style in too long it can also cause hair damage because of lack of moisture.

CONCLUSION

In conclusion, Maintaining healthy hair is important for both its aesthetic appeal and its overall health. To keep your hair healthy, you should establish good hair care habits, such as washing your hair regularly and using appropriate shampoo and conditioner for your hair type. Regular trims are also necessary to prevent split ends and breakage. You should avoid harsh chemicals and sulfates, which can strip your hair of its natural oils and cause dryness. Additionally, heat styling should be limited, and a heat protectant spray should be used before styling.

Eating a healthy diet, rich in protein, vitamins, and minerals, is essential for healthy hair growth. Protecting your hair from the sun's UV rays is also important. Being gentle with your hair can also help prevent breakage, especially when it's wet. Finally, reducing stress through relaxation techniques like meditation and yoga can help prevent hair loss and damage.

Remember that everyone's hair is unique, so you should experiment with different hair care routines and products to find what works best for you. By following these tips, you can maintain healthy and beautiful hair.